Praise for The Lo

Greta Stoddart:

"This is a poetry of learning in the best sense, learning through disassembling, through picking the lock: through opening a lock by using something other than the key - suggesting as it does an unusual, even defiant, method, unexpected and improvisatory as it proceeds; what will I see when I crack this, will I break or open it, what in the end will I see ? Sue Proffitt is a poet of compassion which expresses itself in poems that move continually towards understanding and connection. Nowhere is this more clear than when she 'with one finger, gently' peels back the eyelid of her dead mother to see what it is she sees. And it is this unflinching gaze, this clarity of vision that is both unsparing and merciful, that lends this collection its sense of solace and acceptance.

These poems also show how coping with illness can be a fine balance of drudgery and insight. What the poems are so good at is lifting the moment of reveal from the everyday to ask what - in the positive sense - can be taken from it. Essentially what one receives from these poems is how we might learn from what we have to endure.

There is a great physicality in this collection that seems to run alongside or lead to the spiritual; an interweaving of physical and metaphysical, presence and absence then back again, hope to despair then back again.

Proffitt experiments with form in often surprising ways that present the disorientation and effects of the mind battling to express itself in the breakdown of self.

Mother and daughter find themselves on two sides of an ever-widening gap but still, despite the eventual chasm of mental or relational affinity, there is nevertheless a deep, subconscious bond between them that offers moments of solace and defiance in the face of this overwhelming illness.

A lyrical, tender collection that manages to counterbalance all the strange and difficult truths of witnessing dementia with a certain tough acceptance."

Jane Spiro:
"The Lock-picker invites us to sit alongside the poet as Alzheimers gradually erases the mother she has known and loved. The journey from first diagnosis to its inevitable end is shown with shattering intimacy, taking us close into painful turning points, sharing the very words spoken or scribbled as if we are beamed into the scene itself. What makes the collection so exquisitely tender, is that in this story of loss, the poet reclaims so much of herself: childhood memories, her mother's care 'like a blanket', her own unconditional love as her mother breaks down the boundaries of normality and sanity. The poems do not try to tidy or disguise; they are unflinching in their honesty and their 'refusal to forget'. There are few collections that cover this ground, and in such a way that the reader and perhaps other carers, might feel changed as a result, wiser, kinder, and as Proffitt hopes in her preface, 'a little less alone'."

Alasdair Paterson
What is particularly moving and distinctive about *The Lockpicker* is Sue Proffitt's unerring ability to convey, with a meticulous and inventive commitment to finding absolutely the right forms and language, the encroaching darknesses and confusions of a disintegrating mind. The mother-daughter relationship at the heart of the collection is explored, not only in terms of the grief that witnessing such accelerating loss brings, but also through affecting moments of laughter and rapport and the shared balm of the natural world.

Palewell Press

THE LOCK-PICKER

Sue Proffitt

The Lock-Picker

First edition 2021 from Palewell Press,
www.palewellpress.co.uk

Printed and bound in the UK

ISBN 978-1-911587-47-7

A CIP catalogue record for this title is available from the British Library.

Acknowledgements

The following poems were first published in Open after Dark (Oversteps Books, 2017): 'Skylark', 'My mother's Language', 'Ropes', 'The Night Call' and 'Another Place'. Many` thanks to Alwyn Marriage for permitting their re-publication in The Lock-Picker. In addition, 'Skylark' was highly commended in The Writers Bureau Poetry Competition, 2010. 'Ropes' has also been published in *Artemis, Issue 10*. 'My mother's eyes' won Second Prize in the Teignmouth Poetry Competition, 2018.

Grateful thanks to Hawthornden for their generosity in giving me the gift of time and space in a beautiful setting. This is where most of these poems were written.

Thanks, as ever, to Greta Stoddart and my writing group at the Poetry School's monthly seminars, who have given me so much helpful feedback over the years. Also, 'thank you' to Litmus, a group of poets in whose sparky and stimulating company I've learned a lot about my craft, and to the Company of Poets who have offered insights and inspiration.

I am deeply grateful to Tara Carr for the book-cover; she intuited just what was needed. And huge thanks to Camilla Reeve, my editor, for her patience and constant encouragement.

Finally, my thanks to Julia, for her unfailing support.

Dedication

For my mother Jeannie

and for Anthony and Wendy, my brother and sister,

with love

this collection is also dedicated to the many people

caring for those suffering with dementia –

for your courage and resilience.

"and yes, I know it's you;

and that is where we will come to, sooner

or later, when it's even darker

than it is now, when the snow is colder,

when it's darkest and coldest

and candles are no longer any use to us

and the visibility is zero: *Yes.*

It's still you. It's still you."

Margaret Atwood,

From *Shapechangers in Winter*,

Eating Fire, Selected Poetry 1965-1995, Virago, 2014

Contents

Preface

This is a love story. I remember the day when my mother, Jeannie, was first diagnosed with dementia. It was 2006 and we were sitting in the office of Dr. Wild, a psychiatrist, in Bolton. Jeannie went through the Mini Mental Test as I sat beside her and, for the first time, I confronted what was now inescapable and made sense of the last few months: the worried calls from Jeannie's neighbours to me, the growing sense that something was terribly wrong.

Alzheimer's came into our lives as a strange word, trailing many fears behind it. Once the diagnosis was 'out there', it seemed that everyone who saw me had a story to share about their experience of witnessing dementia. Without exception, the stories were frightening and I used to wonder what motivated people to offload them onto me: in what way they thought such acts were caring. From the outset I knew I would support Jeannie through this illness to the end and said this to her; it was inconceivable that she should go through this alone, as so many people do. This decision was, in part, unavoidable as my brother lives in Australia and my sister had family commitments in Nottingham. But it was more than that. Jeannie and I had had a difficult early relationship. We'd worked hard on healing the wounds between us and had become very close, making up for lost time. It almost felt like a 'given' that I would accompany her down the dementia road; we had a deep commitment to each other.

But I had no idea what that shared dementia journey would be like. I began to avoid people with scary stories, closing such conversations down firmly before they started. Jeannie moved from the north-west to live near me in South Devon and, like millions of others, I began reading up about the condition, trying to understand what was ahead and how we could best resource ourselves through it.

It's now five years since Jeannie died and fifteen since her diagnosis. In looking back over the ten years that she suffered from Alzheimer's, I've asked myself whether I'd have made the same commitment if I'd known then what I know now about the impact of the illness, not only

1

on the sufferer but on those caring for them. The answer is that I would, without question, but I'm glad I didn't know. Not knowing allowed me to adapt, bit by bit, to the changes that occurred in Jeannie and in our relationship. Human beings have an astounding capacity to adapt; we encounter the unthinkable and learn, somehow, to accept it. As we adjust, a new unthinkable thing rises up on the horizon and we learn to adapt to that too. It's a cumulative process; the landscape changes irrevocably around us, and we pause and look back at the land we knew before the illness. But the new landscape becomes what's familiar and slowly we travel through it, without map or compass.

It's taken these five years since my mother's death for Jeannie to return to me in dreams and memories as she was *before* she became ill. Dementia takes away so much: not only the memories of the sufferer, but a significant portion of my memories too. Writing this collection of poems about those ten years has been instrumental in helping me to let go of her illness and to perceive it as something separate from both her and me. In so doing, space has been created in my mind and heart for Jeannie to return. But The Lock-Picker isn't just an act of separation; equally important for me is the need to honour those ten years. That might sound like a strange word to use, but I look back on that time and feel overwhelmed by the courage my mother showed throughout that time, and her unremittingly fierce resistance to the disease.

Jeannie was unusual in this respect; many people with advanced dementia appear to let go of their moorings and drift into a kind of placid suspension until the end. Instead, my mother seemed to retain an insight into what she was losing right to the end and fought it: distraught, inconsolable and frightened for most of the time she was ill. This, more than anything else, was the hardest experience to witness because there was so little anyone could offer her in the way of comfort.

I also want to honour the disease itself because, despite the fact that it is a merciless and terrible condition, Alzheimer's is also a great teacher. I've learned so much over the last ten years, and what I've learned has changed me.

2

Dementia teaches us to be in the present moment: that's all there is, the here and now. All the great spiritual teachings make this point: that the past and future are irrelevant, simply constructs of our minds; all that matters is now. When you love someone with dementia, this is brought home in the strongest possible way because, over time and in Jeannie's case quite slowly, both her past and any sense of a future evaporated. It's difficult to describe how disorientating this can be, as if I was constantly losing my balance. In the early years of the illness, I would enjoy a lovely afternoon with her and the effect of that would trick me; I'd instinctively orientate myself into imagining her as well. 'Imagining' isn't the right word; of course I *knew* she wasn't well, but all the years of knowing her, knowing *us*, when she *was* well, were so much stronger than that more recent knowing. When she seemed to come back to her 'old self' for a while, it returned me, too, to my 'old self': to an 'us' that actually no longer existed. When I got home and rang her, I'd somehow assume she'd remember our afternoon together – would still be in that place. But it would be gone: completely erased. Moments of loving connection occurred and disintegrated and there was no reference point to return to, for her or for me.

The erasing of the past of course includes not only the most recent past, but also, over time, a whole life: everything. Bit by bit it falls away but not cleanly; sometimes it would be as if certain rooms in Jeannie's mind would light up again, and then fall dark once more. Slowly the lights of Jeannie's life – her memories, personality, her sense of identity, switched off. The loss was indescribably painful, both to those around her and to Jeannie herself.

But I learned to adjust, to let go of the past. I learned to move into the moment of being with Jeannie and accept it for what it was: no more, no less. If it was good: a loving connection, then that was a joy, even if a very painful joy. If it was a difficult, painful experience, there was a comfort in knowing that this too would be erased in the next moment – that it wouldn't remain a torment for her. This teaching has changed my relationship with my own sense of past and future; it's helped me to dis-invest so wholly in both.

Of course, everyone's experience of Alzheimer's is different. No two people will be the same, just as no two people suffering cancer have exactly the same illness. During the latter years of Jeannie's life, when living in a bungalow was no longer possible and she had to move into a nursing home, I spent many hours with her there. The whole of the top wing was devoted to looking after residents with dementia, and I came to know many of those residents well. None of them were like my mother.

But I believe there were commonalities in their illness, as there are in the experiences of those caring for them, and that, too, was a core reason for writing these poems; I wanted to write about my experiences as a carer as honestly as possible. I didn't want to avoid the painful and difficult stuff: the intense bouts of boredom I felt, the frustration, the rage, the anguish.

Our relationship deserves no less than the truth in remembering it, and in sharing that truth I want this collection to offer heartfelt support to others going through similar experiences. I want carers to feel less alone: that it's OK to feel these things - it's *human*, and inevitable. Being alongside someone with dementia is, at times, literally maddening; I used to feel sometimes as if I was hovering on the edge of 'losing it'. Jeannie's capacity to lose it, which increased as her internalised inhibitions around what was socially unacceptable disappeared, and there wasn't a remembering of our relationship to hold her back, felt like an invitation for me to 'lose it' too; we could go mad together and then nothing would matter anymore. That's a frightening place to be, and I'm sure I'm not alone in feeling it.

At various points during Jeannie's illness, I recorded some of our conversations. I did ask my mother for her consent in this, which she gave, but I also knew that she wouldn't remember giving it. This was (and still is) uncomfortable for me, but my discomfort is mitigated by why I did it and what the recordings have given to me. Listening to them takes me straight back to the experience of being with her; there's something about hearing all the ambient noises: birdsong, a clock ticking, my mother's beloved cat, that returns me to 'being there'.

This is memory at its most potent, and I needed this to write about my experience. It was also extraordinary to hear the way my mother's brain became so creative as it struggled with dementia. As ordinary vocabulary diminished, she would sometimes come out with remarkable – I want to say poetic – ways of saying what she meant. For example, she once described someone she met as having a 'smile like scissors' which I understood immediately to mean she hadn't trusted him. She would never have said such a phrase when she was well.

I haven't listened to all the recordings; I have about thirty of them. They return me to those years so immediately and powerfully that I'm not ready to hear them all yet. But some of the poems in The Lock-Picker are based around recordings I have listened to, and they bear witness to that time. Despite my discomfort, I'm glad they exist and they have a central place in my remembering.

Being unsparing about the more difficult aspects of caring for someone with dementia means that this isn't an easy read. At times this has made me doubt myself: why am I not presenting the illness in a 'positive' light? Is there a risk that this book will make people feel worse? I hope not. For me, expressing the truth about my experience means there's nothing hidden and, therefore, nothing to be afraid of. Caring for someone with dementia is terrible at times, but that's not the whole truth; there were also moments of grace, moments of connection that seemed to exist outside of time and place, outside of the dying brain. Alzheimer's might take away a person's identity, but what I experienced with Jeannie was the extraordinary power of love as a cohering principle that takes over when memory has largely, or wholly, gone. Jeannie lost a sense of who I was, or who we were to each other; I became different people to her at different times, as her memory flickered and faded. But what was never lost was her awareness that she 'knew' me. When I appeared at the door of her room, sat by her bed or lay next to her on top of the bed and cuddled her, she 'knew' me. She knew my face, even if she couldn't name it or place it. She knew she was safe with me; she knew I loved her.

5

What a gift: in the ravages of dementia something remains inviolate, and can only be called love. I look back now and see my years alongside her as a privilege; there's no greater intimacy than caring for the dying. I wasn't a perfect carer by any means but I did my best, and so did she: that's all we can ask of each other.

As the ground slid away from underneath my mother, I sometimes said to her 'it doesn't matter that you don't remember; I remember. I can remember for you'. I would offer her memories, as did my siblings and other close family members when they visited her. Sometimes she remembered, sometimes not: eventually, not at all. But what I learned was that those who love the person with dementia become the 'holders' or 'guardians' of who they were, when the sufferer can no longer do it for herself. In writing about my mother's last ten years, I'm refusing to forget; The Lock-Picker holds my memories and, inside them, they hold my mother. I hope that in reading them, you come alongside us and, if you're in a similar position to me as a carer, I hope this book helps you feel less alone.

MISSING

"You come back into the room

where you've been living

all along. You say:

What's been going on

while I was away?"

Margaret Atwood

from *You Come Back*

Eating Fire, Selected Poetry 1965-1995, Virago, 2014

Short-circuiting the crow

Anxiety stalked you all your adult life
the crow on your shoulder
only a crisis could explode

like when I fell down the stairs
years ago, boiling coffee
flying sideways,

something snapping
inside me
inside you –

black feathers whited in the blast –
you lowered me to the bedroom floor
rang the ambulance

got a blanket
lay down beside me
to keep me warm

while we waited.
So calm.
Short-circuiting the crow.

I had never known you
such a mother as then
when love was a blanket

you pulled over us.

Missing

Something's missing
where is it
something essential
necessary as breathing
your address, where is it

you reach back to that place
where it always is,
you reach back with your hand
without looking
(you don't need to look)
to that place where your credit card is,
your cheque book, your tickets, but –

what are these numbers
you've written here
over and over –

this question you've started
to scribble but not finished –

and this, this thing
what's it for –

before, you could reach back
without looking to that place,
that passageway in your mind
swift and smooth as an oiled chute,
as a slide down a banister

but now your fingers flail,
grasping at air.

The Mini Mental Test

Dr Wild. The first.
Taker-away of your driving licence –
unforgiveable deprivation.

Overall picture moderate
to low. Definitely some decline.
Scan shows slight shrinkage.

For the first time –
possible Alzheimer's?

Remember these three words
in this order. Boot. Purse. Poppy.
I'll come back to them later.

I'm doing this with you
in a neutral room, under
the silent regard of the clock.
Name? Yes. As you struggle
with your address, name
of the prime minister, what year it is
I answer for you silently.

Boot. Purse. Poppy.
I push a red poppy's petals inside
your small white purse, lock them
in the boot of the car
you can't drive. There.
Ready for you to retrieve.

So can you remember those
three words I told you earlier?

No. Your eyes, bright, frantic,
gaze at hers, your little laugh
that will slide to a sob
when we're back in the car.
Here they are!
Wrenching the boot open,
pressing the purse into your hands,
without moving. *Here they are!*

Breaking the news

The first person you tell
is your best friend

when we get home
the house indifferent

humming its hot water tune
under its breath

heating the living room
where you sit with her.

I see you
from the hallway

hear the diagnosis,
your voice tentative

the way you might say
a foreign word

ignorant of its meaning
your best friend saying – gently –

at least we know now
what we're dealing with.

She died weeks later –
catastrophic absence

you could not conceive
any more than you could see

the face of your illness
or understand

how it would learn to speak
through your mouth

turn all your thoughts,
words, foreign.

Where's Bunny

Now that you have gone
I can return to the story –

how you turned up on the doorstep
of your friend's house asking for her.

Where's Bunny? you said,
white strain on your face

the effort of keeping at bay
that dark slick lapping at your edges.

Where's Bunny? I don't know
how they – grieving, baffled –

answered you
but somehow the words were said

Bunny's dead. Bunny's dead.

This is the part I find hardest –
the sudden hit: a crumpling inwards

your mouth open,
inchoate anguish of sounds

and how, when you turn to leave,
the terror is there in your eyes

because you see it now for a moment
how you are falling in on yourself

before you're there again the next day
with the same question

all knowing erased.
The story plays itself out

on my closed eyes – your open mouth,
the bright hopeless question.

Skylark

Let's stop, you say.
We get out of the car into Summer.
The lane dreams bees
in a blue ache of sky,
a humming filigree of flowers.

Listen, a skylark! I say.
Excitement brightens your face
like a child swinging open
the door to an empty room,
singing.

We look up -
see the blurry-feathered dot
swallowed in light,
a down-shimmer
of disembodied song.

You stand, holding the car-door,
smiling.
The moment has come
(I never know when it's coming)
side-stepping you

out of illness,
washing you in its urgent beauty,
                    now, now –
I watch you
brought back by a skylark.

A Problem

What goes out
fades at the edges first,
the way a fire does.

Here is a fireplace, look.
Full of black stones.

Somewhere
you remember
what to do.

The engineer is worried.
My mother is picking up the phone

over and over again,
ordering coal
for her 'living flame effect' gas fire –

she's lighting them with matches.
Gas pipe underneath.

I've disconnected it.
Later this week
the coal merchant

will remove the coal.
Problem solved.

Home

In the time of small things
    losing themselves

bits of paper torn
    from notebooks

words scribbled without
    beginnings or ends –

in the time of cooked fish
    in the cupboard

cornflakes
    in the fridge

when my phone fills
    with thirty-two messages

from you
    what shall I do

when everything was
    a *muddle* –

a ballet, film,
    shared meal

could still bring you home
    to yourself,

needing to know
     I was home too –

don't forget to ring ....
     let me know you're back safely

Bullseye

Within my mother
a formless fear rises
and I interrogate it
as if I can call it to attention
make it state its name,
reason for being here
label it 'irrational'
then line it against a wall and,
bringing my mother out to watch,
shoot it.

As if I can.

As if I do not know
that the bullseye
is behind my mother's eyes.

Your diary

You pore over
its arcane map
of numbers
and scribbled words:

Tumbly Hill
coach picking me up
making   unmaking
crossing out   repeating

the torch you take
into the black cave –
flickering intermittent
spotlight

on   what?

The dark doesn't answer.

Footnote: *Tumbly Hill is a day centre for the elderly and infirm.*

A nice evening

They still happened
but rarer –
the odd shining light
at sea.

At yours. You're happy.
Back. Sweet animated chat –
*who would you like
to spend the day with?*

Someone said *Shakespeare.*
Joan of Arc for me
and you said
David Attenborough!

In he came,
into the room
into your brain
known and smiling.

Oh my heart
what would *you* have said
if asked – for a whole day –
you, mother, you.

The Map-Maker

I am the cartographer of madness –
blank spaces   fraying ends
      snapped threads
              lanterns cracked.

I draw the maps that remember
countries my mother walked
which disappear behind her –
the vanishing lands.

I mark out the graves
of her forgotten selves,
sometimes trace an archipelago –
each scattered islet

a memory intact   but adrift –
I trace the rivers
that plunge underground
without warning.

I am the compass-bearer
searching for my mother's hand
to guide her to the map-edge,
let her go

In this story

it is always Summer when the birds
have forgotten endings. The sky is brilliant –
falling through the long glazed pane of the window

into the living room where the daughter
laces the heavy hooves of prescription boots
to the bird-bones of her mother's feet.

Here they come now
through the back door
around the side of the house

the mother is grasping at pipes
at mortar at rails at her daughter's arm
as the alien paving stones beneath

her alien hooves pitch and slide.
They sit at the table that knows them not.
The mother, hunched in her carapace

of blankets and cushions,
looks inwards where there is ruin.
The daughter lifts her face

to the sun but something crying
drags her back from bright air and birds
who don't remember endings

No brakes

Impossible, not to turn child with you –
mowing your front lawn
decapitating wild geraniums,

your face at the kitchen window
gesticulating –
mad mouth moving in rage

one hand flailing
Come in! Come in!
So hard not to stop, obey.

You were never stern.
Why can't I ignore you?

Something inside you
knows no limits
now.

Something has reared up
shouting.
Something inside me

hesitates before your face –
is afraid
because there are no brakes.

Still frame

If I could I would stop it here,
outside the front of your house.

Late afternoon sunlight
stroking your hands

holding a trowel, planting pansies
in the bed you could reach

without bending. In their tray
purple and gold faces

and *your* face, lifted up, smiling
as I drive away.

CRACKS

"A suffering you can neither cure nor enter –

There are worse things, but not many.

After a while it makes us impatient.

Can't we do anything but feel sorry?"

Margaret Atwood

From *Flowers*

Eating Fire, Selected Poetry 1965-1995, Virago, 2014

My Mother's Language

In the early morning, as the tide pulls back,
her first sounds wheel and fidget on the foreshore

getting their bearings: *where-why-what*
pick-pick of scavengers tearing at weed,

turning over pebbles, throwing up a crab-claw,
hunting for the left-behind

titbits in the dislocated kelp
flung on the tideline.

By lunchtime she knows, like the gulls,
there is something there under the flotsam

of discarded cups, a tangle of ropes,
a bloated shoe, each half-known thing

unearthed carefully, held up for an instant
to the light —— and dropped.

What is that unrecognisable thing
out on the water? Under a million stones

small words scuttle out of sight,
and out of the frightening sky

a cloud-shift quenches the afternoon light,
makes even the shallowest pool

impenetrable. In the puddled sand
a mystified calligraphy of webbed feet

circles the same phrases over again
and she reaches the sea

more by chance   — sinks down
under the waves' heave.

Ropes

Summer, sun pressing against the window:
a child denied attention.
The fire is on, 'The King and I'
choruses its story.

Do you remember?
lobbing memories like ropes
begging a catch.
Yes I do!

Your smile returns you
so that even now
six years disappear –
singing *Getting to Know You*

as I knead the bumps
and cracks in your feet,
resting in my hands
like broken birds.

And I wonder who's clinging to whom –
you, grasping at the parts
of yourself I throw towards you,
or me, watching

your frantic eyes go under,
scrabbling in the wreckage
for something, anything
to keep you afloat.

By every bedside
in every airless room
so many, half-in, half-out,
flail beseeching hands

and those of us on the edge
hear our voices pleading
let go! let go!
all the time throwing ropes.

Ghost Talk

(from a recorded conversation between my mother and me)

My mother: Did she say kicking today...
Me: The carer said you kicked her yesterday. Not true?
My mother: I don't know... I think it's true... I don't know what to do.

(Silence. She cries.)

Me: I think you should apologise when she gets back.

listening in on us
like the ghost of Christmas Past.

I'm reading the paper – hear its angry flap –
silent in the face of your crying

monotonous as a dripping tap
a hiccup that won't stop,

the mercury-bubble of my spirit
dropping slowly by degrees

down the funnel of your misery.
My ghost-self sees clearly

you don't remember kicking anyone.

Useless to feel sorry now
to wish I might move the paper away,

in my ears whisper

remember – she can't remember.

*This will end, and you want
to recall how bad it was.*

*Not only for you though
Not only for you.*

My voice

pitched at one tight note
does not deviate

no matter that my mother hacks back
what is strangling her

pulls out a branch still green
though cut and offers it to me.

Olive. I can't see it, receive it,
instead crash about

in the kitchen. Sit her down.
Feed her. Criticise her.

This is the territory of failure.
Easy to say if I could

I would pause it.
Instead I replay my voice –

its hard white glaze.

Grace moments

We pick up with each other
as easily as if you had just left
the room for a minute –

here you are: sweet smile,
ready laugh, *known* again –
my animal-knowing *home.*

I never think *how long will this last*
or even *I miss this*

instead, in the warmth
of your sun's random return,
close my eyes –

soak it up, the full-flood
of *ordinariness,*
those millions of moments *before*

it breaks.

Occlusions cross your face, words
stutter in the shift and slur
of something retreating –

the dark's back.
I watch
our slow obliteration.

What shall I do my mother says

her fingers knot and unknot
picking at something.

There is no answer to this.
There are a thousand answers

but only if you consider it a question
like her fingers question

knotting and unknotting
no I don't want a drink

pushing away the mug of tea – it spills –
something's leaking away

what shall I do
a wail emitted like the siren

of an ambulance stuck in traffic,
fingers picking and unpicking

looking for gaps between log-jams
small clear spaces

underneath the plaque
accreting layer upon layer.

Her fingers fretwork the air   if only
if only   something could be unpicked –

neurons flowing freely
across synaptic highways

to their end –
she pushes away my hand

flip   stick   knot   twitch
pick   unpick

open mouth   un-minded
neither moored   nor un-moored.

The betrayal

It isn't the body that betrays itself.
It does what it does.

Here, in my mother's bedroom,
I pause at the open drawer
of her bedside table

and somewhere in the corner
watch myself making the decision.

Now I see myself telling her
something unspeakable
but I can't look directly at her face –

what must have happened
to her body, stiffening in recoil,

throat slamming shut
how her mind must have frozen
bringing the thick blind eye of ice

down over this knowing – *are you sure...?*
I can't believe....Maybe someone else....?

while two neat parcels,
wrapped in toilet paper, lie mute
as sarcophagi inside her drawer.

If I had known then what I know now,
how each *betrayal of herself*

levers open her fingers' grip,
I would not have shared that betrayal –
leaving my mother alone

on her bed, the crush
of morning light on her shoulders.

Cracks

October glows blue in your eyes
      where cataracts slowly   crystallise, unseasonal.

Your bedrock shifts.
      Cracks – hairline at first –   deepen, split

this is the ground now

but still I whisper in your ear
      about the librarian's skirt   cement the cracks –

make you giggle – in the bank
      steady you enough   to write a cheque

but I never forget

we're on cracked ground.
      Dark opens under you   in the dazzle-din supermarket,

we run from it, laughing
      at your illegible   shopping list

meaningless words

jumping cracks one last time –
      please god   the ground holds

when you sight an egret
      on the estuary.

So funny

What is it about laughter

               when the unbearable hits me,
               lurching sideways

suddenly into your madness?

               That time you twisted
               the skin slowly –

chinese-burned my arm –

               we circled like two boxers
               in the hall. *Let me go!*

Into the night in your nightie. No.

               Looking down
               at your hands, all bone,

so resolutely hurting me

               I could feel it
               bubble up

refusing

               to believe –
               so funny

or that day when

               I left the shop –
               you were in the car –

and, returning,

               saw your small bum
               tipped bare

out of the half-opened door

               weeing down the street
               I could feel

my mouth falling open

               inside –
               you,

so shy

               so ladylike –
               so funny

My mother wakes up and thinks it's morning

Slurry dark, blind as wet wool.
Something orange sliding across the wall.
I'm in this bed which is mine,
I know this. My head on the pillow.
Aching in every part. My feet
are broken. Get them, get them
off this bed, onto the floor.
Here it is. Clutching mattress,
bed-head, now I'm standing.
There's the door – it's morning.
Head for the light
under the door.
Open it. Hallway.
There she is – I know her face
but my throat tightens
her expression says

> there's something
> wrong
> with me

No, not morning yet,
you've had a doze. It's night now
crooking her hand under my elbow
and it slides, all slides away
I don't know anything
where I am what time it is
my mouth opens in an O –
she will fill it with tea.

Three voices

(from a recorded conversation)

She gasps like a dog run over, panting in the road,
or as if she is running, running, to get away

but the orthopaedic chair lifts her flotsam body
out   up   into the air   suspended

where she speaks

It's worse when I'm like this.
You've got it all.
I've forgotten most of it.

My voice is on auto-pilot.

You have nothing to be scared of.
You're quite safe.
What do you mean, you don't know where you are?

Liar voice.

In the silence the cat mews,
un-listened to.

My mother needs me to be frightened.
Instead, I put the quiche on.

The Night Call

Your mother's upset
the carer said on the phone.
I can't get her to bed.
So I went. It was about nine at night,
the cul de sac was quiet,
lamp-lit, all the windows closed.

When I walk in, my mother
is circling the hall, shaking off
the carer's hands. *They're out there*
she says, *my children,*
all alone and it's night.
They're only young. Let me go,
let me find them.

She pushes away my soothing arms
and my words fall off her.
Around and around she circles,
struggling for the door,
brute strength
in her desperation.

Back in the car, I dial her landline
from my mobile
and there, in the waiting dark,
a tiny-child voice grows out of my throat.
Mummy? I say.

I tell her we are all right —
staying with our Daddy —
we'll see her tomorrow.

Her voice quietens.
Are you sure you're safe? she asks.
Yes, I reply
and sit there in the silent street
where, at the edge of the street lamp's glow
our three small shapes —

brother, sister, me —
stand just out of sight.

Hope for Suee

(written in my mother's shaky handwriting in a tiny notebook, undated)

SUE ENERGE
SUE ENEER
ADULT PREES
PLEE LEA
HOPE FOR SUEE

I see her bending
over the table

resting the notebook
on something hard

biro pressed
into little crab fingers

something hard
to write

remember

the effort it takes
to hold that thought

clear, finished
CAPITALISE IT

feel it fray
dissolve

disintegrate
try again

and again
something so hard

HOPE FOR SUEE

was this my name
          me, for a second?

My mother's secret voice

(heard on a recording)

I too have a secret voice. It comes if I'm lonely
or frightened; the tide's strong, I'm not making headway
swimming back to shore –

there it is, flowing out of my throat
(emphatic like a parent) – *you can do it*
there, keep going. Now, I hear yours.

When was it born? After diagnosis, I guess.
How the pressure must have grown –
what you can't show –

'*Would you like a cup of tea?*' I ask, disappearing
into your kitchen. *Yes please!* you say brightly,
and under sounds of tap, kettle, clattering crockery

your secret voice takes its longed-for chance to speak –
I don't know what to do, what shall I do, oh god ....

The moment I'm back in the room, it goes quiet.
I don't know it's spoken: opening up – sickening –
your life swerving, sliding, out of control.

Little terror-voice, low and guttural.
I have to turn the volume up to hear you.
Little hopeless voice, croaking to the cushions, to the cat,

who listens and knows. *What shall I do?*
Hearing you, years too late, I'm silent.
Now, as then, there's no answer.

Your secret voice knew that too.

Hoovering

In the days when I make sounds
for the sake of it
when accepting silence
feels like failure,
I visit my mother one grey afternoon.

In the bedroom, the carer flails
a hoover, smiles and waves
a memory of my mother in –

> *a corridor of dusty sunlight.*
> *My mother is pushing the vacuum cleaner*
> *up and down, its long bag a sail*
> *in full wind, her foot pressing*
> *its secret pedal*

I walk into the living room.
My mother is half-tipped
off her chair gasping
face wet and contorted
mouthing words I cannot hear
over the sound of hoovering –

> *at the end of the corridor,*
> *she turns, smiles at me*
> *presses the pedal off –*
> *afternoon sunlight fills*
> *with lavender floor-polish*
> *and my lego-boat is free again*
> *to sail the long ocean of corridor*

The lock-picker

is at your back all the time now
caped in the kind of night
that is starless. Faceless.
Such an intimate embrace.
His hands are fine, long-fingered,
the fingers of a jeweller.
Lock-breaker. Thief.
He uses silver tools
to un-rivet, unscrew,
dis-assemble. It is hard
but he is patient,
he has all the time in the world.

Your mind does not want to die.
It flickers and spasms
at its un-fashioning –
flares up, all windows blazing,
then out – half-out – a dull glow.
Being prised apart so slowly
is such a subtle death. Held
in his embrace which is extinction,
what a press there must be
to surrender. Fall back,
leave the doors open.
Let him at it.

ANOTHER PLACE

"The days are gone.

Only one day remains,

the one you're in."

Margaret Atwood,

From *A Visit*

Eating Fire, Selected Poetry 1965-1995, Virago, 2014

Mrs. Proffitt

You moved into residential care
to 'try it out' – hated it.

All I do is sit in a chair all day.
I can't make my own meals.
I can't wash my own clothes.
I don't even have a cat to care for.

You couldn't do these tasks
on your own
but *Mrs. Proffitt* was – still –
the face you knew in the mirror

so I moved you back.
It took another year before
sitting in a chair all day
no longer mattered.

Nursing Home, 10 pm

shouting

screaming

whispers

even at night
a ruckus
from one room
to another

laughter

ricocheting
through walls

banging

or small-spore
whimpers
multiplying

threading themselves
along corridors

questions

repeating repeating

the mycelia of
the sleepless

a bleep
signalling
which room
where

singing

your no-place
no-time
besieged

crying

Moving into the nursing home

Picture of a toilet
on the bathroom door
dementia-friendly!

Your name on a door.
I stick photos under your name:
your room!

In the corridor wraiths totter
frail as bleached twigs.
A woman rummages

through a chest of drawers
deliberately unlocked –
they like to rifle through ...

beads, bracelets, buttons,
odds and ends –   .
makes them feel at home ...

on the walls, posters – 1920s, 30s –
postcard souvenirs
of far-flung places

Get on the Orient Express!
Summer in Brighton!
Picnic at Kew Gardens!

Doors open and close.
Your door slowly
edges open

a man shambles in,
puzzled, looking at us.
not in here ....

my firm voice ushers him out –
you, shocked into silence
by invasion –

a nurse enters.
There you are Michael,
come with me ....

    ... sorry about that.

Full Circle

Look, you have a nice room!
All your things in here,
your own armchair
your own bed
pictures on the walls.
See your clock?
It's yours, from home!

Don't cry. There's nothing
to cry about. Soon
the trolley will come
with tea and biscuits.
Even your own mug!
The one with the cat on it
remember?

Please stop crying.
We can have tea together,
meals too,
and when I come back –
soon – we'll go for a drive
somewhere nice
something to look forward to!

You don't have to see
anyone. This is your room
with your name on it.
You might make friends
Rosie in the room
next to yours seems nice
I know you don't remember her.

You'll get used to it,
the staff are only
trying to help
and look! You can see
the garden outside!
When I come back –
soon – we'll sit out there.

My bright, implacable voice –
your voice –
leaving me at boarding school.

The residents

Betty. Rake-thin. Bright-eyed.
After mealtimes up and down the corridors
                    managing the pub she ran for years
in and out of rooms   tidying sorting putting away
stops me in the corridor
holds my hands
gazes intensely   *I'm so busy!*

Bill. Wheelchair bound.
Slumped as a half-full sack,
a slop of food down cardigan and shirt.
Slurred speech, rheumy eyes
sparking at any interest   *you're a good girl*

Jill. Irascible crow in her chair
one black coffee allowed a day – no sugar –
showing me the photos –   *I was in the oil business!*
Middle East, smart suit, smiling.
She has a son in the navy who visited once.
There's a dress she loves, wants to show me.
Later I say – and the moment's gone.

The stick-arm protruding from the top
of the cot in the room opposite
shouting out the tuneless childhood song –
                de dah dah de dah dah de dah dah!
                de dah dah de dah dah de dah!
over and over,
full of rage.

The woman who never speaks.

The man who smiles – hits out –
can't be left alone.

The woman who's blind
calling calling all day long   *help me!*
her voice echoing down the corridor

cadaverous forms hunched on beds,
vacant faces turned ceilingwards

    -    in Room 30
        one face

Treachery

Just one spoonful more
you won't remember
the last one
was the final spoonful.

You'll enjoy it outside
wheeled around
a strange planet
rigid under your blanket.

It's not so bad

but it is.

I'll be back soon
knowing that as the door
closes behind me
I am erased

and the flood
drowns you.

Occupation

In your room
where nothing happens
hour after hour

captive, desperate,
I turn to newspaper, book, phone,
even the tree that moves, that speaks,

but every time my eyes turn away
you haul me in – hooked fish –
pull me up on the deck

of your beached boat
its rotting timbers
open holes

ripped sails,
there
to stare at you.

My compulsory attention –
it's how you feel
yourself alive –

occupying the space
in *my* face.

Standing guard

A continent has erupted in your face
purpling eyes, nose, cheek bone
and my rage hurls itself down the phone line.
You sent her in an ambulance alone?

We are cubicled in A & E.
You shift, recoil from voice, touch,
foetal under a sheet.
It's two o'clock in the morning

in an alien hive, criss-crossed
with stretchers where a line
of small curtains flap open, close,
each concealing its crisis.

A hubbub of voices, machines,
and that peculiar cocoon
not-even-half
illusion of privacy

curtained-off –
as if this plastic membrane
can do what your skin
no longer can –

protect you.
Things happen to you now.
You have no agency
over events –

the tray slips,
the floor slides
the orthopaedic chair
falls away as you rise

and the ground slams
you hard
contusion to contusion.
I am your guard

stationing myself
ferocious
by your side.
Too late.

I enter the ward

My mother walks towards me
down the aisle.

So you've come at last have you?
I suppose you've come from HER?

The hinges have blown loose
from the capsule of my mother's mind

and now we land anywhere.
The door to her face bursts open

and I don't know who
will be in there –

what role waits for me.
I step forward into my father.

You, father, abdicated long ago.
Your second chance,

if you want it. No matter
if you want it or not.

Mother – something raw whips
out of the door

round the bones
of your face –

66

show me what you hid,
how it hurt.

Let me say
I'm sorry

My mother is turning bird

Her fingers' uncut nails
        lie on her lap. Small talons

waiting to strike at proffered pills
        glass of water or a pessary.

At the Raptor Rescue Centre
        inside a dark recess, something flapping, tearing.

I peer in. Wild eyes stare back.
        Peregrine trussed by the feet jerking itself

to the end of its short runway
        of rope again and again.

Nailing down a winged thing.
        I stop breathing –

the closest I get to that feeling.
        My mother doesn't struggle

doesn't even turn her head
        but her body knows what violation is.

Readies itself.

Snake-Strike

Holding your hand in the corridor
outside the staff room, this could be school –
parent meets with teachers –
quiet chat about meds, the challenges of care
that ducks lashing-out nails.
You small and silent beside me

then your fist in my face – snake-strike fast –
hard, hitting its target without you
even looking, child in a nightdress,
your rage a white concentrated heat
from which I pull away
reeling.

Two years later I see it –
that stunted coil
of comprehension
deep in your brainstem's dark
suddenly alerted –
itself *being talked about.*

Another Place

In this room time slows
to the drip drip
of tea, biscuits, pills

advancing trolley wheels
the discreet knock,
an endless bleep.

A torpor, thick and heavy,
anaesthetic, seeps through me
but not you.

You drag your distress
to the edge of the chasm
at your feet

over and over again,
waking me up to see you,
dark silhouette

framed in panic's bright filaments.
My reassurances drop around you
useless as dead birds.

But there is one way
to bring you and me
to another place.

I take you to bed,
watch your slow collapsing
bone by bone,

a litany of whimpers
bringing you close to my side.
Now, sometimes,

we can sleep at last,
the wisp of your hair's drift
on my cheek, your sour breath

suspended in the air
like a blessing.
I hold your hands. Wait.

The question

Stepping into your room again –
its failing light – I remember, now,
                    what you said before

will you do it?
The ragged grey heron
                    I want to die

flew uselessly around your room
returned to roost inside your throat
                    but this time

something followed. You threw out
the line from your sinking boat –
                    would it catch?

I answered as you might expect.
The hopeless close
                    of your face.

I have betrayed you many times
but never more than this,
                    knowing –

in that moment – how often my eyes
have moved from your eyes
                    to your pillow.

Your parents

You say they're waiting for you *upstairs*.
Two old people

mute and anxious. Faces concealed.
How do they

hear you? How do you hear them?
The way you know

someone's listening at the top
of the stairs

without looking. Or your ears
hear your mouth's

words spoken aloud on the air –
suddenly separate.

Lost child. They're listening
to you calling.

Squatter

There was a time
when something animated you
that was not you.

I don't mean the rages
or when memory was a box
burst –   detritus

we could not pick up
we could not put back
into order.

This was beyond that.
The box had gone
or maybe

it was still
on the floor
irrelevant.

I mean the time
beyond lost memories
beyond voice

when you were eyes
watching but I don't know
what you watched

when you were bone
surfacing. When it was
hard to approach you

look at the strange planet
of your face blowing out
its gases

and yet. Something in you
knew me. Was it your soul
I saw briefly

stripped of what's human –
all the cladding we drop
into when we're born?

A squatter
caught at the open window
of a condemned house?

Easter Sunday 2015, nursing home

One last time
you open your arms
wide as heartbreak

Susan!

My name and not my name.
No matter.

When you stroke my arm
this is real.

What lovely eyes you have!

You look at me.　　　You　　look　　at　　me
a whole field of flowers in your smile.

How lovely you look!
I love you. I love Brian too ...

My dead father.
No matter

because it's time now to make it all better

the floor is falling
under your feet
and the house is burning down –

a good man. A lovely man really.
Go outside and see him.
Give him a kiss.

I move seamlessly
between realities –

words are snakes
shedding skins –

you've been seeing
your mother, your father. Both said
nothing much.

My mother walks with the dead now.
I don't go there!

As good as.
Her dead self speaks freely.
When I leave can I come
and stay with you for a while?
That would be lovely.

I can't believe we have lived
ten minutes
where you only smile,
hold my hand –

where there is only love
in your eyes,

all the souls of your family
passing through you

permeable as fog   *Oh it's nice to see you.*
retreating seawards   *See you on holiday!*

77

Knowing

Nothing else to look at except the window,
        sitting by my mother's bed. Early evening.

I have no idea where she is or what it is
        that breathes, still. Her eyes are closed, something

has come down between us which is final. I cannot enter.
        And if I could I would not lean into her face turned towards me

inhale the reek of her breath. Her body is engaged in its
        business of extinction, great swathes of cells switching

off. What do I do? We're both in suspension
        but my mother is busy. *How long* whispers

the treacherous thought. Then I see the vast cedar
        in the carpark flashing white lights, black branches explosive,

snaring a sinking sun. Dark agitation, off-beat lighthouse,
        flares from a boat at night – and I know. The knowing

sinks instantly, embedding itself on that edge
        inside my eyes for six hours before it awakes

                                      ignited.

Her memories

I will never know the rest –

you and your younger brother
in a Bedfordshire field, crouching
as the German bomber flew low
over your heads

I want to ask

*What were you doing
in that field?
What happened next?*

Now

The dying are not senseless.
On the edge they wait
alert as a wolf

for the moment.

The wrecked body hums,
its black box
flight recorder

on the ocean bed

not sending out
signals –
receiving them.

room   empty
corridor   quiet
daughter   gone –

now!

pulling out –

for some,
one look back
at what is on the bed.

ORPHAN

"You spiral out there,

locked and single

and on your way at last,

the rings of Saturn brilliant

as pain, your dark craft

nosing its way through stars.

You've been gone now

how many years?"

Margaret Atwood,

From *Out*

Eating Fire, Selected Poetry 1965-1995, Virago, 2014

Orphan

A new thing –
childless
parentless.

Something young
in me stops
considers –

fingers to mouth.
No one behind
or before.

Waking
in the pre-dawn dark
I see

the DNA twist
that is me:
uniquely

threaded stems,
flowerheads
of cells

spiralling upwards
through
the empty

architecture
of my body
to its end.

Mirage

On the nights my mother appeared
to the night nurse after
she was dead

I believed

in her bell ringing in an empty room –
that she might sit on church steps
with an armful of tulips, smiling

revisit people, places

for the last time.
I have seen the ghost of a rainbow
hover in soaked air

after the sun vanishes

alchemical bow
imprinted on the retina
for an instant.

Behind soft white ash

why not for one heartbeat
extended, her eyes,
smile, her shining hair?

My Mother's Eyes

When I opened my mother's eyes
I expected glazed windows.
Deep fog through windscreen glass.

It was a troubling thing to do.

They weren't completely closed
but even if they had been
I'd have done the same

in those hours just after –

that terminal silence
when clocks still go
and the medicine trolley rattles

its mad monologue down the corridor

but in this room, nothing
but the dead-bird body
of my mother

I think I did it to make sure.

No. I knew.
But the one unbroken line was between our eyes –
when everything else had snapped

one look – tiny isolated spark –

still jumped a connection,
wordless, nameless,
memory-less.

Was it still there?

With one finger, gently,
I pulled each eyelid up.
There they were –

blue still, clear, fluid.

Were they empty?
No. They held the look of someone
leaning back into the body of a mountain

looking down

Curl

I knew I was going to do it –
take the scissors, cut one curl
from my mother's head

in the silent time
alone in the room
but not alone –

the window open
a pearl light
pouring over us

bringing bird song,
early-opening petals –
she hovered

curious I imagine
moved by my rituals
watching the prayers I whispered

undulate and shimmer in the air
above the sunken husk
of her face

but her hair remained
the same. Just behind her ear
a new-born's curl

silver and springy
wraps round my fingers,
pushes back against my press

to straighten it out.
Now it's in a locket.
It's far too heavy

for what it is. I took death
with it when I cut one curl
from my mother's head.

Inside the locket

A web in the corner
of a church window

fluff half-pulled
from a bird's nest

eye, filmed
in floaters

what's snagged
on barbed wire

unravelling. Something
slowly darkening –

her ancestors
compressed.

A spring, still,
when I touch it with my finger.

Breath

I am looking for my mother in the caves of the dead

        how they open backwards
        how the dark sucks itself

and I follow
knowing only the soft press of heel on stone

        nubs of toes
        another step
           another

                    drawn on

as if the dark is one long in-taken breath –

sometimes
in this room at night

        I am in a lidless tomb
        staring up

                and wonder
                when I turn over
                facing the wall

if I'll hear her   behind me

                exhale

Here is my mother

Here is my mother, inside me.
A compression. Ten years
bound tight as cord
round raw meat.

But this is the thing –
where is she *before*?
Nothing moves past the window
where I look out for her.

You know the story.
A woman listens for the ghost inside the house
but it is outside that a figure
passes by the window.

Nothing reads my name
traced on the foggy glass
or watches the searchlight outside
moving its hard white disk –

random, useless – across the years.
Absence is milk-white.
A bowl I put my finger in
again and again,

feeling for the

How she is with me, everywhere

Animal tracks in the snow.

What shall I do?

Do this. I stalk, try to decipher, follow prints into the deep slush –
                                      broken twigs, buried leaves
where they stop.

Everything is a muddle

I know. Stories interrupted, so many lost. The river drives
                                    itself downstream,
not counting its losses –

I feel funny. Life isn't much fun anymore ....

My foot slips, slides down the unseen bank
                                    crushing snowdrops.
I'm looking for the grey dipper
its flare of gold on ice

not much fun for you, me tagging along!

                                    but it's not there.

A mess of tiny leaf-shreds under birch – deer's thin pickings –

what shall I do?

Do this? I press my hand again and again
                                    into a tree's white stump –

fingers, touching.

Black Hole

There isn't one of us
that hasn't a black hole
in that silver bowl
of the mind –

a throat intent
on swallowing –
too small to see,
lightless.

In the Milky Way
a vast one
lies in wait.

You forget it's there
until one day
up ahead,
you spy

the miasma
of your life
rippling
a ragged ring

around something
unseen –

its bright tatters
like children
dancing
mesmerised,

downwards

It is two years now

and I am tired of carrying
your dead outline
inside mine

the grey bloom
of your illness
on my heart.

Kneel and look.
Listen to where
it is crying.

Lift the heart out into salt
the cold spring wind
the indifferent surge

of the tide
pulling away
moss-cling

leaving –
if I shift mud
with my foot –

wet space
shining.

If you were here

I'd say *Walk?*
You'd say *I'm game!*

We'd step into sun
                              not enough, yet,
to roll back snow's white hood

though fern-tips of pines rise
delicate as black feathers
pricking the sky's diffusing shine

            – and one bird throws
three small flutes across the gap
between window and rock

            calling itself to the question

on the other side,
each note trailing its bell-echo
in space

            as our voices would

            – half-heard phrases
a laugh catching the light
                              bright, untranslatable –
in the gaps between trees
as we climb, unseen

Last words

These things are mine, I said
I will cradle them as carefully
as a small bird. Some are buried
but it doesn't matter –
I can feel them without looking.

These things are yours:
cloudless blue
with or without a smile.
Something hurt and half-hidden
in a forest.
A handful of wild flowers
stretched for through a car window.
The tissue of old letters
not expecting a reply.
A pock-faced doll.
A flattened cushion that spells
long sitting and waiting.

And these are ours:
a body of water.
An open fire watched.
The moment before stepping out
when anything is possible.
Talking late into the night.
A door pushed open
outside everything known.

They're still there, I said.

On the anniversary of her death

Silence is no more still than air,
thundering through space like a river.
But if I listen to it in this room
it stops – attends – as all things do
when attention turns, regards them.

Into that silence I say
I would do it again.

Behind the vast grey fog of your illness
was the black sun where all light enters.
I could not know this
until its shadow had passed
over my face and moved on.

I walked with you for so long
that we knew ourselves only
by the faces we became –
until I could not find you
though I called –

no one could have fought harder.

We might spend the next life together
saying *sorry* for this one
but there was no practice run
and you and I, so bruised,
made a pact of sorts –

never once broken –
to see it out.

I saw you out. Now
I release the river
from its held spell –
it roars away through dark rocks
underneath this room.

Sue Proffitt - Biography

Sue Proffitt – www.sueproffitt.com – lives by the coast in South Devon. Her poetry explores the beauty and mystery of the more-than-human world, and of our complex human relationship with it. She has an M.A. in Creative Writing from the University of Bath Spa and has been published in a number of magazines, journals and poetry competitions. Her first collection, Open After Dark, was published by Oversteps in 2017. In 2018 she was awarded a Hawthornden Fellowship and it was during that month, in a snow-bound castle outside Edinburgh, that The Lock-Picker was born. She is currently working on her third collection.

Palewell Press

Palewell Press is an independent publisher handling poetry, fiction and non-fiction with a focus on books that foster Justice, Equality and Sustainability. The Editor can be reached on enquiries@palewellpress.co.uk